How to stop watching porn

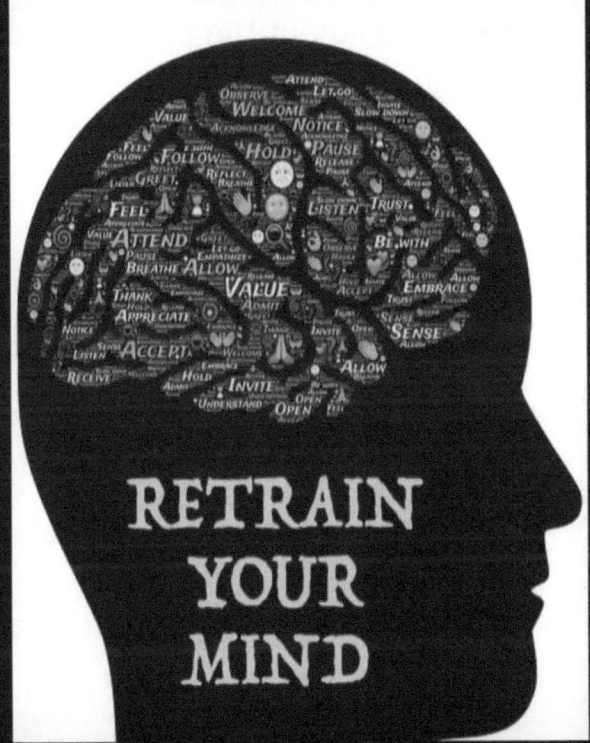

RETRAIN YOUR MIND

Do it yourself tips and techniques to overcome porn Addiction

Ethan J.George

All Rights Reserved © Ethan J. George

All rights reserved. This book or any part of it may not be copied, edited or re-written in any format whatsoever without the permission and approval of the Author.

How to stop watching porn

TABLE OF CONTENTS

Introduction..1
Focus..2
Mind Control Techniques........................3
Workout..4
Socialization...5
Overcoming Porn Secret Tips...............6
Eye Technique...7
A Partner..8
Therapy and Counseling.......................9
Addiction Support Groups..................10
Religious Beliefs...................................11
Conclusion...12
About the Author..................................13
Disclaimer..14

INTRODUCTION

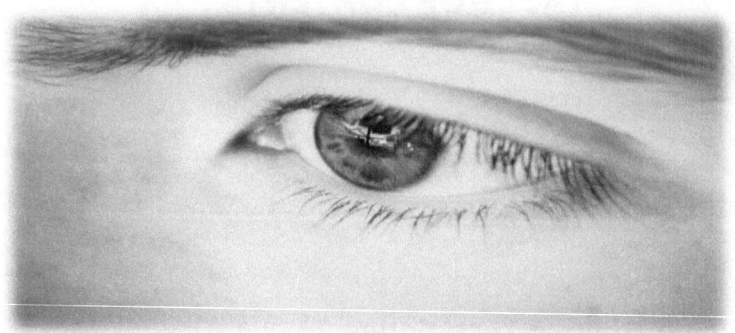

Pornography often referred to as "porn" is a representation or depiction of sexual behavior with pictures, status, by using media, like print materials and videos for sexual excitement.

It was an English word used in the 19th century, a Greek word known as (pornographos) which means the act of writing or displaying about prostitution which is meant for sexual amusement and arousal.

Ethically Pornography is seen as an immoral, noxious, addictive and termed illegal with obscenity laws and mostly censored by government of most nations globally.

Negative effect of pornography this days greatly has to do with models who take photographs being nude or half naked and porn actors and actresses who engage in acting films or videos clips performing sexual intercourse known as blue films.

However it will also be interesting to know that such acts are more tolerant in the western world thereby making this videos easily accessible by kids, teens and adults to continually come across pornographic materials online, magazines, videos and animations

It will interest you to know that the first blue film was made by **Andy Warhol**, it was full of erotic display depicting sexually explicit intercourse which was released in the United States of America.

Internet and home videos in the 20th century brought about a boom in the consumption and production of pornographic videos which generated billions in dollars for porn industries worldwide.

Commercially today porn accounts for US$2.5 billion in United States of America, and the year 2006 saw huge revenue in porn industries worldwide accounting for 97 billion dollars and it has giving jobs to thousands of people who act and company staffs who are responsible for filming and recording it.

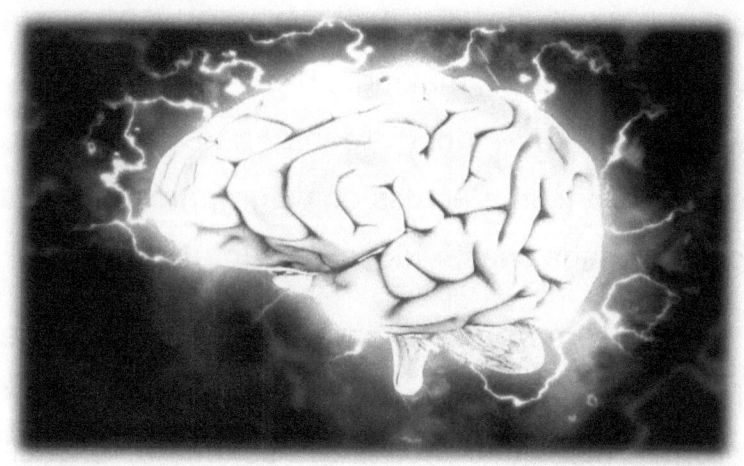

There are millions of online and offline materials both soft and hard copies circulating everywhere you go today globally and millions of sites hosting pornographic live performances and acts.

Pornographic content consumption has been found to be addictive, cause's depression, erectile dysfunction and distortion of neural wiring in the brain, it has a very strong trigger which can make the brain to change and still adapt which is known as plasticity.

In the future continuous watching of porn will lead to natural sexual dysfunction, such as trying to achieve an orgasm and erection with a human partner, it makes the human brain to be wired to respond to sex stimulation with the help of dopamine in it.

Porn has caused allot of problems for those people who are addicted to watching it all the time and has developed poor mental health condition and low 2level of living standard of lifestyle, it's compulsive which makes you keep wanting more of it and also affects once brain mirror neurons and that can lead to sexual violence with your partner physically.

Porn watch is known to damage a human's brain region which is responsible for making decision, acting morally and impulse control, so as a result it damages your prefrontal cortex and makes an individual to take poor decisions that will affect his/her life negatively.

Porn may appear to be helping you quench your sexual urge at a point but if you really know how it has been twisting your brain on making life decisions and at a point you become miserable and hopeless as a result of negative effects of porn on your life then you will realizing it causing you more harm than good.

Watching porn lead you to do so many bad things such as masturbating each time you watch it, raping someone or a minor and abusing any female close by,

It's believed that most school shooting this days by high school kids is as result of porn messing with their brain and substance abuse as both of them mess up your brain and compel you to do anything once you're under their influence.

FOCUS

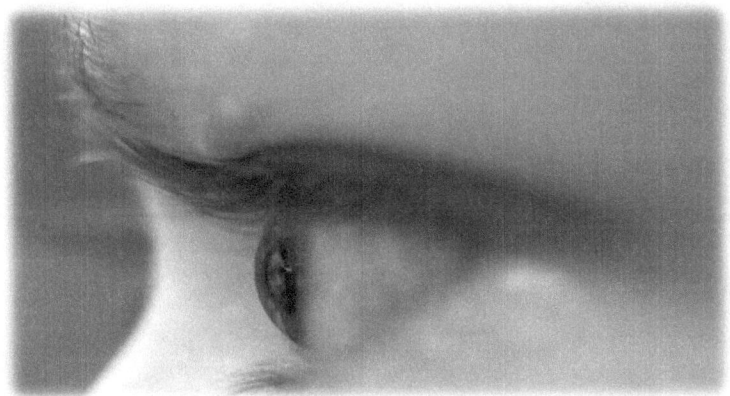

In life when you want to start something new which can be a habit, change of lifestyle and improve on yourself, there is a level of seriousness you need to practice and adhered to for you to be able to keep up and never relapse, Which will include persistence and constant practice of your new lifestyle for you to be able to achieve your desired goal.

You need to have a road map within you with a vision of what exactly you're up to and try to maintain it even with allot of distraction and temptations come but if you're serious you will see yourself there in less than no time.

Since you have made up your mind to quit porn it can be achievable if you are focused and follow a path which you believe and achieve it, make sure you obey the rules at all times and retrain your mind so that your body and spirit can have the willpower to conquer temptation squarely when the triggers comes.

You will have to sacrifice some things of pleasure in your life for you to be able to refrain from porn, it's not just been vocal about it, you will need to take decisive actions such as reducing the level of watching TV, using internet and stay away from things that generally will make you come in contact with porn or nudes.

Porn is compulsive so for you to quit you need to gear yourself up by resisting it each time you are tempted to watch it, you can sleep off, leave the room and go and sit outside, play a game, take a walk for the urge to pass, you will need to sacrifice allot of things to keep up and not relapse and go back to it.

MIND CONTROL TECHNIQUES

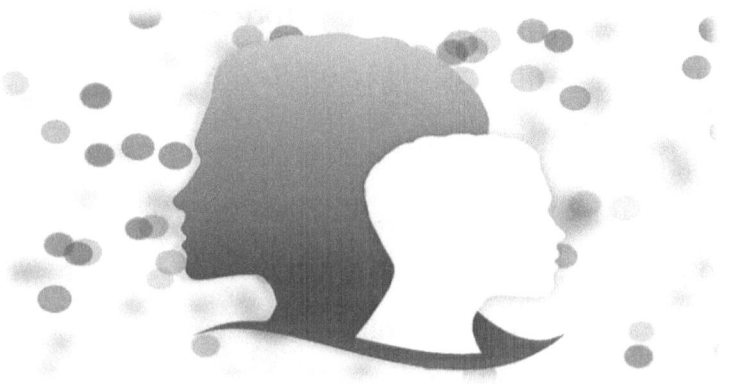

Umans beings are double minded which can be positive and negative thoughts, the positive represent acts which bring about good things in our lives when we act upon them and the negative thoughts which can leads us to self-destruction, but it's a human beings ability to maintain self-discipline and control the mind towards working towards the positive side to leave life ethically as required of us all.

Any act or decision you take in life the mind always way the both options before you can take a decision and at this point not minding the consequences that may come up later, funny enough no one cheats nature, so bad decisions always have a future repercussion which you will face later on in life.

Pornography Watching is a disgusting act and when you're addicted, it becomes part of you, makes you lazy and unmotivated to do any meaning stuff that will bring progress in your life, it's unhealthy and leads you to allot of problems psychologically, morally and physically in your social life and body as well.

It's well known that addiction to watching porn makes you act inappropriately in work places, schools and other events you partake in, it's compulsive most especially when the urge comes and continues watching leads to chronic masturbation which is very unhealthy to your body.

Porn addiction affects your brains neural wiring and makes you behave abnormal and it has some certain control over your life which may seem spiritual, but it's far from that as scientist have proven how it can rewire your brain to change and adapt to its ways of pleasure easily, so that it will constantly have control over your life.

Mind control towards porn addiction has allot to do with pictures or images your eyes have captured and sent into the brain for interpretation.

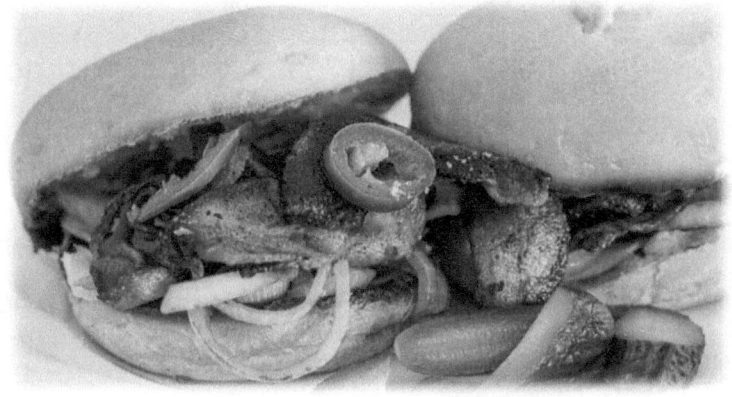

How this technique will help you is by getting images of junk foods from the internet and viewing them 3 times a week so that when you come across porn anywhere it will be as if you were looking at a junk food and it will be disgusting to you. Try doing this for 3 months to get better results.

Mind control has to do with your inner thoughts about porn, if truly you want to do away with it, you must admit within you that you have an addiction problem and also make up your mind that you want to get rid of it, since it's impacting negatively in your life and be prepared to sacrifice allot to stop it permanent so that you can leave a normal life.

How your mind control porn triggers is not easy but it can be controlled by distracting yourself using instruments like guitar, piano, drum etc. the time you investing in playing an instrument has finish you will realized you no longer have the urge to watch it anymore.

The mind is the Centre of the human body so it's an area you will need to give a serious attention for you to be able to stop porn addiction and live a fulfilled life without been compulsive as a result of watching porn.

WORKOUT

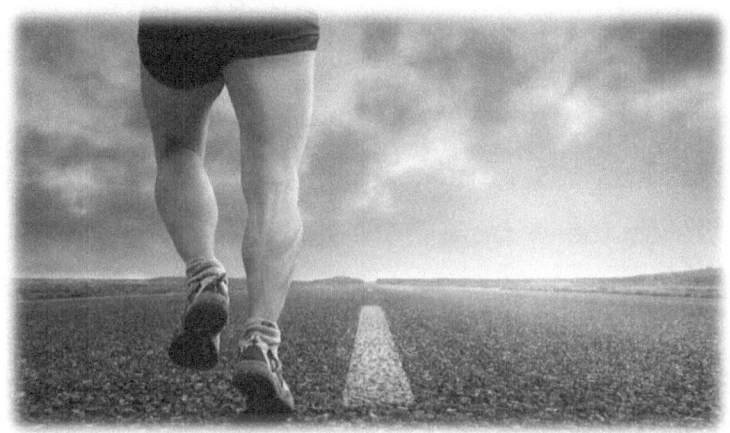

Scientific research has found out that watching porn continuously depletes the chemical in the brain which is responsible for pleasure called dopamine.

Workout which are mostly light exercises can help re-charge and replenish dopamine levels in your brain so that it can withstand impulses such as porn addiction.

When porn depletes the dopamine level in your brain it leaves you unmotivated, depressed, unfocused and lethargic, they are well known as porn watching triggers.

When you do exercises they will help the levels of dopamine baseline to increase which then motivates new brain cells called receptors to grow which makes you focused, motivated and also fight porn addiction, you will gradually be able to loose from porn compulsion and start to think and act properly as a normal human being should.

Recommended exercises can be light walking and performing yoga which can help you allot in rising your dopamine levels, it's also advisable you stand up frequently most times within the day than just sitting for long hours all day.

The technique here is that standing up most times within the day will serve as a form of light exercise to raise dopamine levels so that you won't have much time to sit down and watch porn, being up makes you keep yourself busy than sitting all day.

SOCIALIZATION

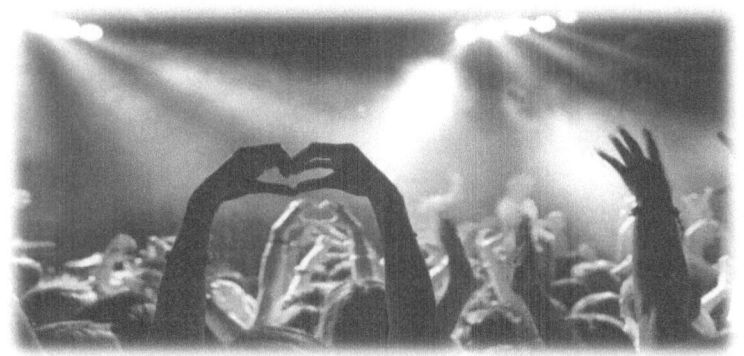

Watching pornography is not only dependent on TV or online, it can also be referred to display of nudity by modern girls who dress seductively and half naked in the name of modern fashion which can be termed as physical porn.

Whether it's been displayed along with the male counterpart together having sex or not, there is highly display of private body parts by modern females this days that should be covered for decency sake.

Social lifestyle has to change as well for you to truly overcome porn, there are places such as nude parties, drinking joints such as brothel with a lot of prostitutes and strip clubs where allot of sensitive body parts are been exposed constantly by entertainers and stripers.

Its paramount you stay away from such areas for you to fight and overcome porn addiction and you won't be tempted to go back into watch it again, so make sure your eyes are constantly not coming in contact with this seductively or half naked dressed girls or entertainers.

It's said bad manners corrupt good ones, so it will be nice to avoid or stay away from your porn addicted or sex chats friends who can't go a day without talking about sex and who watch allot porn, because the more you stay around them you will won't have positive results on your porn addiction recovery journey.

Neuroscientists have said when a brain accepts any bad habit it can never be wiped out from your memory completely, but there are two things you can do to bring it down to a minimal level which is by not giving it the opportunities it must have to operate and by staying away from those things permanently.

And if you can learn to override it with a more pleasurable and healthy habit that will make you to be glued to it and then never go back to the bad or unhealthy one that has become a problem to your life.

Travelling out of your comfort zone where you stay and watch born helps you cut down on watching porn when you leave your immediate environment and go on business trips that keeps you busy working.

After travelling it will be wise to keep yourself busy by working on a particular project or goal so that you can be able to take off your mind on watching porn.

It's believed boredom is one major reason why many people involve in the watching of porn so by keeping you busy and moving from one location to another will totally reduce level of watching it and gradually coming to a stop.

OVERCOMING PORN SECRET TIPS

There are daily tips which can help you overcome porn addiction, so we are going to categorical list them here for you, then advice you on how to go about them yourself physically, so that you can be able to free yourself from porn addiction permanently.

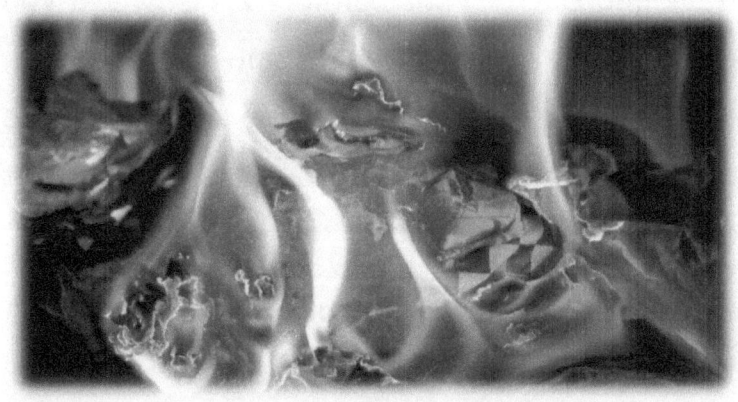

Burning digital and print materials; these are electronic devices and print materials such as books, magazines, erotic novels etc., they are materials filled with so much pornography that we always come across on daily basis, and be tempted to look at them or watch or read.

Most examples of are devices are mobile phones, PDAs, Tablets, IPod, computers with other electronics such TV and Disk plates (CDS).

They are virtually everywhere as we live our daily life and we consume them so much it becomes an addiction especially the ones with pornographic content and it becomes unhealthy.

To become a new person you will need to take a drastic action to leave this kind of lifestyle, which you probably have been living for years. So at this point you have to be focused and have the willpower to maintain your stands on leaving porn, so that you will be able to live a normal healthy life.

First and foremost clean your house, office or place of work with this print materials, by burning or incinerating them as the case may be.

Then you can move on to the devices by which earlier mentioned, like in the case of TV there is always a family parental control button to block channels showing pornographic content, which you can have someone who doesn't live in your house to come and lock it, with a password that none of the family members will know about it including you.

Same password method can be used for your online devices such as phones, laptops and computers when you download site blocking soft wares or apps. Let him or her not review the password details to you so that you won't be tempted to access them.

Try to stay away from stores where you can have access to this materials, so that you won't be tempted to buy again when you go there to get something.

Be focused and take this measures seriously and you will see your life changing gradually, and you start engaging yourself with serious life issues which initially it kept you away from.

Habit loop Hack; it's one of the highly recommended working technique to use and gradually overcome an addiction, porn which gives so much pleasure, is replace with a hobby similar to it.

Something that you're always motivated to do and can't get enough of it, so replacing it with something you love doing subsidizes the porn addiction.

It can be physical exercises, sports, napping, working on a project and selecting a TV program, to replace channels and programs showing porn content and from there you will start forgetting about it gradually.

It has rewired your brain, so it will take time for it to clear from your memory, and that can only be a gradual process, if not you will relapse and go back to it.

Make sure whatever you choose to do is something that you feel fulfilled, it's enjoyable and also keep you busy so that it can replace the time you used in consuming porn.

Just make sure it's something that your passion about and always be consistent, so that your brain will be reset to such events and no longer porn.

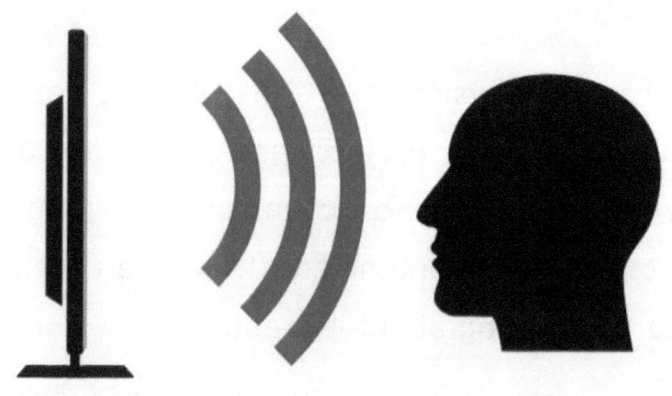

Identifying addiction origin; try to rethink on how you started watching porn, it's possible from there you can know the reason, why you started in the first place and with that you can find a better way to work on yourself to overcome it.

From research, highest percentages shows that most porn addiction problems started is as a result of boredom, drifting away of partner, easing daily stressors from work places, mostly jobs where you are been stress up with allot of work.

It's advised that some of the issues listed above, if you can resolve or reduce them with the lowest minimum, there are likely chances watching porn addiction will gradually come to a stop soon or someday.

As for boredom, you can decided to schedule each activity you intend to do on a daily basis to keep yourself busy, until it's sleeping time then you will go to bed without viewing porn in a whole day.

Whenever you have a relationship problem with your partner, try to work it out, so that as result of you not having sex for long, you won't be tempted to console yourself with porn and ended up picking more interest in it.

Porn addiction can be solved with lifestyle changes, which will have been talking about here or getting a new job to keep you busy, volunteering to help others out, so that you can stop watching porn and live a naturally and healthy life.

There are stressful jobs many people do in a day, which make them to have less time for relationships or resting properly, they end up watching porn to ease stress and overcome sexual urge.

There are simple ways of solving issues like this, such as cutting down the number of jobs you do in a day to reduce stress, and try to get into a relationship at least on, so that you can gradually kill the porn triggers

EYE PREVENTION TECHNIQUES

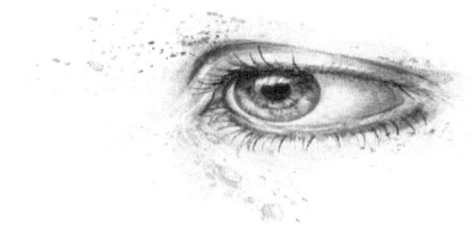

D***igital lockdown***: it's a process of replacing all your gadgets with others without capabilities of displaying videos and graphic images, like in the case of phone.

It's advisable to use a non-camera phone, which will not contain video files for you to be tempted to watch video content. In that way it will reduce or stop your free access to viewing any form of graphic or video content.

TVs also play a very big part in the process of watching porn frequently, especially the one in your private room, because you can access to it all the time when alone, so you will be tempted to watch all the time.

My personal recommendation here is that you should take the TV out of your room or disconnect it, and be using the one in the living room with other people, so that you will hardly be alone to tune porn channels.

Try to watch it mostly when others are watching as well, because if you're alone even in the living room, you can as well use it for watching porn, especially you're head of the house. A situation whereby you leave alone just disconnect and unplug it.

Computers and laptops; It's very important for you to prevent videos with nude scenes especially movies or short porn videos to be stored in your laptop or computer,

So that you will not be tempted to watch them, at this point most videos in your possession should be educative or work based videos so that you will not be tempted to watch them when you're alone.

Body positioning; it's a process whereby you try to avoid things that will make you come across porn or nude, so try as much possible not to be where you shouldn't be, to avoid been triggered, you must learn to avoid this places at all cost, so that you will not easily come in contact with porn.

If you visit someone and the person is watching a program which contains nudes, it will be best you to excuse the person and wait outside or someplace else for the person.

In your personal office, it will be nice if you take out the TV or discount it permanently, especially during this trying times, when the porn issue has reduced to a certain level you can reinstate it.

If you're seating next to someone in a bus, train or anywhere at all, and he or she is watching videos that are exposing too much nude that can trigger you, then it will be nice to simply change your position or seat to another area.

PARTNER

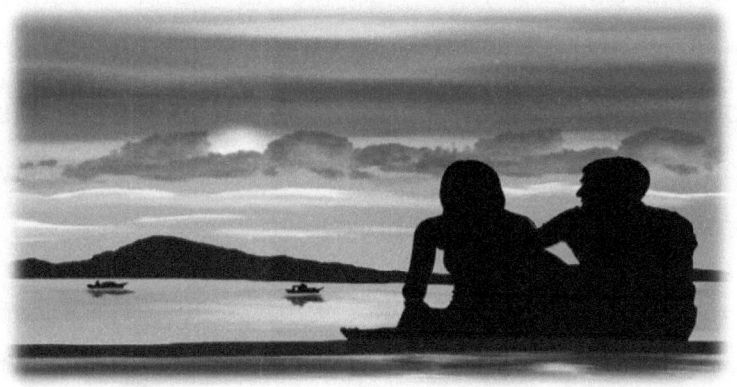

One of the solutions to overcome porn addiction will be getting yourself a female companion, so that whenever you're having the urge to watch porn you can tease your partner and have sexual intercourse together.

both of you can actually arrange on the number of times to have sex in a week or month so it won't be like your using her as sex toy.

Apart from just having sex most of the time with your partner to reduce your urge of watching porn, some of this partners can support you mentally and physically in your healing journey, by talking to you about it and trying to make sure you change from such attitude.

Most people have gone into marriages for the sake of sex addition, porn or masturbation problems, it however turned out to well for most people, but it's not advisable if you're not capable of getting married, then you go ahead to marry because of this issues, you might regret later.

A good wife will be very active to assist in any way possible to stop the husband from porn addiction, virtually all women are unhappy and get jealous if you keep on watching it.

They don't accept it because to them it feels like form of cheating, insulting, degrading their personality, some even go to the extent of ending a relationship or divorcing you, if you're not willing to make enough efforts and stop it.

Some women take out their time to look for a therapist for you, some will force you go if you're not been serious about it.

Some even accompany you there to make sure you are been serious, though not all of them can do that, some will endure it for few months or years and if you don't stop they will simply quit the relationship or marriage as the as may be and move on with their lives.

THERAPY AND COUNSELLING

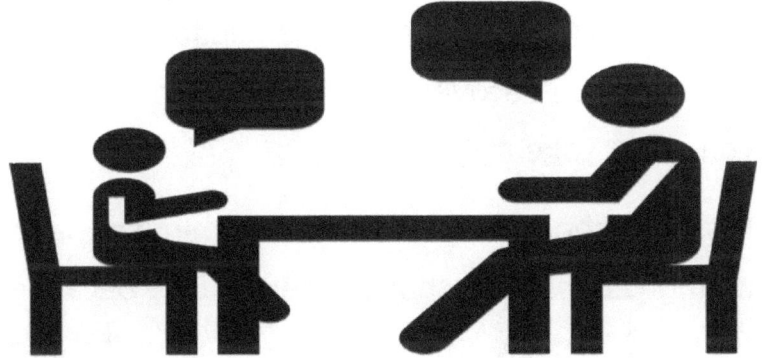

There are lot of licensed sex therapist and counselors this days, that specifically specialized on issues of sexual addiction and recovery you can rely on them to work on yourself so that you can be able to quit porn addiction.

The most important thing is that you will need to take it seriously, because most people don't even go there as scheduled or after registering with a therapist, sometimes its due busy schedules from work and go about their other activities.

There are also people who will don't believe in therapy or counselling, they advise you that it's not going to solve your addiction problem to make you recover, so if you listen to them you won't take it serious.

It's all about an individual's mindset and willingness to stop that matters most, because allot of people have seen therapist and counsellors in the past, allot of them came through so you too can do it using one.

Most of them are trained professionals who use (CBT) cognitive behavioral therapy to treat their patients or clients, they tell you about how your thoughts are being irrational,

Detrimental and how the consumption of pornography excessively has prevented you to live a meaningful life for years, they will train and coach you on how you can have a positive mindset about your sex life and maintain relationships then taking your mind off pornography.

ADDICTION SUPPORT GROUPS

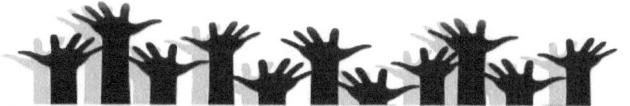

Addiction support groups are all over in any in America and every community have it, if you have an addiction problem, try and locate them to register as a members and start attending meetings.

You can Google it to find the one in your local area to join and become a member, people outside United States which such things are not in their countries or local area can do it online.

It's a place where people suffering with one addiction, or the other come together to share their experiences and learn from each other, on ways they have being handling it and how to overcome it, they learn from each other especially the ones who are applying certain techniques and methods and are getting better results, they have a leader who lead them and give instructions on how to handle issues, you can learn and build on it as well.

The benefits of this support groups are abundant and they will help and guild you towards your addiction recovery journey, in this place you can have mentors who are going to hold you accountable, if they see that you're not being serious about your recovery, and they will encourage you to sit up.

When you become a member, there is this feeling within you that lets you know that you're not alone, it helps you work with other members and come out stronger, most especially if you hear or see physically other peoples condition getting better, you will equally want to see some positive changes on yourself, it will become like a challenge to you.

During difficult times in the fighting process, you will have people who will advise and talk to you most especially if you have tried everything but you feel it's not working, they will teach you conquering tips other things to assist you become better.

There're allot of support groups out there for different purposes depending on your type of addiction and level which it's affecting you,

The most popular ones are known as alcoholics' anonymous (AA) and 12-step program, this ones are mostly for people with higher addiction problems with alcohol, drugs and smoking e.tc.

There are other ones that strictly deal with addictions, responsible for handling emotional problems, example the smart recovery program, secular organization for sobriety, rational recovery, women for sobriety.

They handle things such as thoughts, emotions, to be motivated, learning how to manage urge when they come and how you will be able find to strike a balance to overcome your addiction problem.

RELIGIOUSBELIEFS

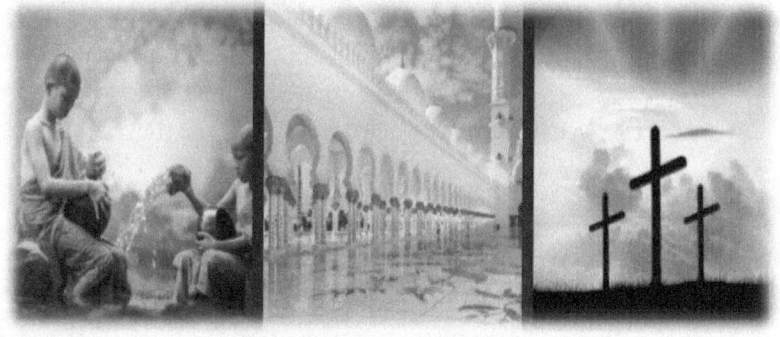

Religious beliefs are ways in which we practice spiritual self-discipline, they are there to guide us spiritually, so that we can act in a positive manner, with an ultimate power will believe in and worship to help us solve our problems.

When we are dedicated to the teachings we receive from our places of worships, it makes us to have faith in ourselves and pray to the ultimate power we worship known as God by Christians.

Prayers coupled with our beliefs in the ultimate power God, help build our spiritual life and inner strength to tackle personal problems with porn addiction, teachings from this worship books such as Bible, Quran etc. out rightly condemn this immoral acts from this religious books.

They have explained how sinful and harmful watching porn or any acts related to it is not good to human beings who have been created for a much higher and better purpose in life.

Praying, fasting and being dedicated will motivate you to change, the doctrines are there for you to read and be guide, to avoid sinful acts and become pure in the eyes of God.

It's spiritually believed you have been associated with an evil spirit which is compelling you to watch porn, you will deliverance from God or the ultimate power you worship to be freed.

That's the religious explanation which is different from the scientific one earlier explained in the introductory part of this book.

CONCLUSION

Pornographic addiction is a very dangerous habit no one should be addicted to, because it will mess up ones brain and it will result to you always losing focus on important things in life.

It's simply a bad habit that can be replaced with a good one, it will only take time but you can overcome it sooner or later, self-determination is a key factor, just make sure you're serious and committed to the lifestyle changes involved to change and it will work.

Everything is centered on your mind and emotions, it you who willingly started watching porn and its same you that will have to change your mind towards it, tips in this book will help in assisting you to stop, but it can never be 100 percent.

Once you work on your lifestyle changes and finally make up your mind you surely overcome porn addiction.

ABOUT THE AUTHOR

Ethan J. George is a publisher and writer who have been writing articles on health niche with many years of experience, and have also added his personal experience on some of the addictions problems he had in the paste, which he overcame as a young man while growing up.

DISCLAIMER

Tips and advice here on how to stop porn addiction are strictly for information purpose and should not be mistaken for medical report or otherwise.

If you have a serious health problem with porn addiction kindly consult your medical doctor for professional treatment and diagnosis.

How to stop watching porn

All Rights Reserved © Ethan J. George

www.ingramcontent.com/pod-product-compliance
Lightning Source LLC
Chambersburg PA
CBHW030518220526
45464CB00006B/2859